A GUIDE TO DEMENTIA FOR CAREGIVERS

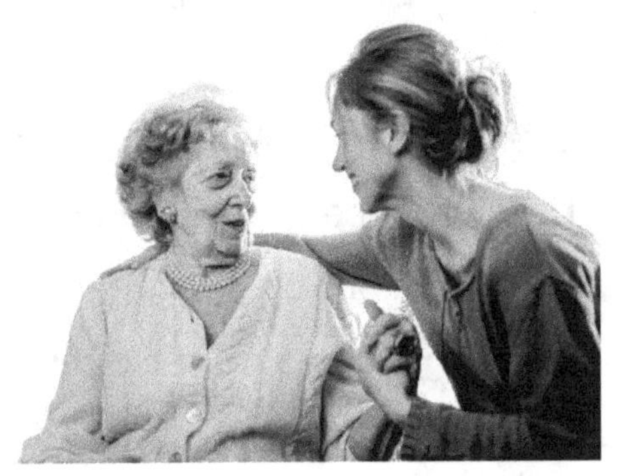

A Comprehensive Guide for Understanding and Managing Dementia Care

Ashley R.Whitlow

Table of content

Introduction

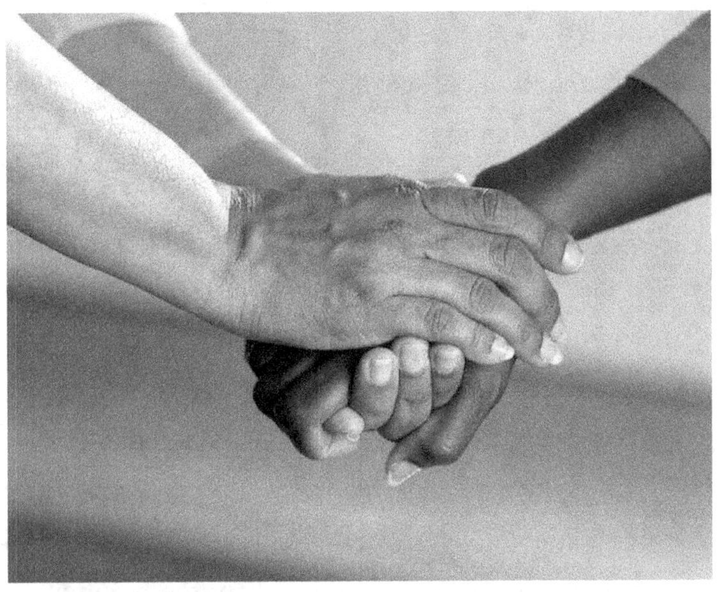

Once upon a quiet autumn evening, Sarah stumbled upon a dusty old bookstore. Curiously, she browsed the shelves until her eyes rested on a book whose title was Dementia Guide for Caregivers. As she flipped through its pages, a new-found understanding blossomed within her.

Provided with the knowledge gathered from the book, Sarah's neighbor, Mrs. Thompson, became the unexpected beneficiary. Mrs. Thompson, once a vibrant soul, now struggled against dementia that seemed to tighten its grip with each passing day. provided with newfound understanding, Sarah approached caregiving with patience and tender-heartedness.

Through gentle guidance and creative engagement, Sarah found joy in the simplicity of shared moments, Sarah discovered that caring for Mrs. Thompson wasn't a frightening task; it was an opportunity to create beautiful moments in the tapestry of a fading memory. The challenges that once seemed insurmountable transformed into opportunities for connection and shared humanity.

As the seasons changed, so did their bond. The wisdom from the book not only made Sarah a capable caregiver but also enriched her own life. In the quiet corners of caregiving, she found the flexibility of the human spirit and the enduring power of kindness. And so, within the pages of the book, Sarah not only found guidance but also discovered the in-depth beauty that arises when caring becomes an act of love.

Taking care of a loved one who has dementia comes with special obstacles that often call for empathy and logical thinking. With the help of this book, which offers advice and techniques specifically designed for caregivers, we set out to go through the complicated conditions of dementia care. As we explore the complicated nature of this illness, our goal is to give you the knowledge and assistance you need to provide effective and compassionate care.

This book is an extensive guide meant to assist caregivers on their way to improving the quality of life for persons living with dementia. It covers everything from knowing the details of dementia to offering helpful guidance on communication, legal issues, and self-care. Come explore with us the importance of caregivers in the lives of people they care for, as well as understanding and adaptability.

Understanding Dementia

A deterioration in cognitive function that hinders a person's capacity to carry out daily tasks is the defining characteristics of dementia, a complicated condition. It is a collection of symptoms linked to a number of underlying causes, the most common of which is Alzheimer's disease, rather than a distinct illness. It is essential to have an in-depth knowledge of dementia when providing care.

Recognizing the early stages of dementia is the first step towards treating it. Initial symptoms may include disorientation, memory loss, and trouble solving problems. Knowing these details as a caretaker enables you to intervene promptly, which may reduce the person's decline and enhance their quality of life overall.

It is easier to adjust care techniques when dementia care are divided into groups. Alzheimer's disease, Lewy body dementia, vascular dementia, and other dementias have different presented traits. Comprehending these distinctions allows caregivers to modify approaches that target certain difficulties linked with each kind, fostering a more customized and efficient caring encounter.

Understanding how dementia affects one's emotional and cognitive health is essential to understanding dementia. Dementia patients may exhibit mood swings, personality changes, and trouble communicating. Patience, sensitivity, and the creation of successful communication techniques are necessary for navigating these transitions.

Establishing a nurturing atmosphere becomes crucial. Making little changes to daily routines and making sure safety precautions are in place at home may improve the wellbeing of both the dementia patient and the caregiver. This section of the guide delves into possible steps for creating a safe and relaxing living environment.

Caregivers will learn about medical care and treatment choices, legal issues, and the value of establishing a strong support network as we look into the complexities of dementia. Caretakers may positively influence the lives of those they look for by approaching their work with knowledge and compassion, provided they have a thorough awareness of the complex nature of dementia.

Types and Stages of Dementia

There are many forms of dementia, and each has distinct traits and causes. The most typical kinds consist of:

Alzheimer's disease: This is a degenerative brain disease that causes behavioral abnormalities, cognitive impairment, and memory loss.

Vascular dementia: Impaired blood supply to the brain, often as a result of strokes or other vascular problems.

Lewy Body Dementia: This is an Abnormal protein deposit in the brain that manifests as motor symptoms, cognitive alterations, and visual hallucinations.

Frontotemporal dementia: This kind of dementia affects the brain's frontal and temporal lobes and causes alterations in language, behavior, and even personality.

Mixed dementia: This type of dementia Combines characteristics of many dementia types, most often vascular dementia and Alzheimer's disease.

Stages of Dementia

As dementia advances through stages, its symptoms get worse with time. Although each phase might change, a basic structure consists of:

Early Stage (Mild): Minimal influence on everyday functioning and mild cognitive impairment with sporadic memory lapses.

Moderate (Middle Stage): Notable reduction in cognitive ability that interferes with day-to-day functioning. Confusion and memory loss become increasingly noticeable.

Severe (Late stage): Severe cognitive decline, physical incapacity, and reliance on others for daily care characterize the late stage (severe). It gets quite difficult to communicate.

Caregivers must be aware of the specific type and stage of dementia to customize their care, provide the right kind of assistance, and improve the overall quality of care for those afflicted with this complicated condition.

Common Symptoms and Behaviors

As the condition worsens, a range of symptoms and behaviors become evident that indicate dementia. Caregivers need to identify these symptoms to provide appropriate assistance.

Typical symptoms include:
Memory Loss: One of the main symptoms is forgetfulness, particularly about recent or significant events.

Cognitive decline: it's the inability to understand, solve problems, or carry out routine duties.

Communication problems: include stuttering, repeating sentences, and having trouble following and contributing to discussions.

Mood Swings: People suffering from dementia may go through phases of sadness, anxiety, and anger.

Disorientation: This might manifest as difficulties recognizing individuals, losing track of time, or becoming lost in familiar surroundings.

Impaired judgment: This includes making poor decisions, being unable to evaluate risks, and having difficulty with planning.

Change in personality: Behavior and personality changes that can be upsetting for the person experiencing them as well as their caretakers will start to surface.

Aggression and agitation: irritability, restlessness, and even physical violence.

Delusions and hallucinations: Believing unfounded things or seeing things that are not there, which may lead to further perplexity.

Sleep disturbances: A disturbance in sleep patterns, such as excessive daytime drowsiness or insomnia.

Caregivers may better prepare for difficulties and adjust their approach by being aware of these signs. By reducing the burden of these symptoms and modifying activities to the person's capacities, supportive environments and effective communication techniques may provide a more responsive and caring caregiving experience.

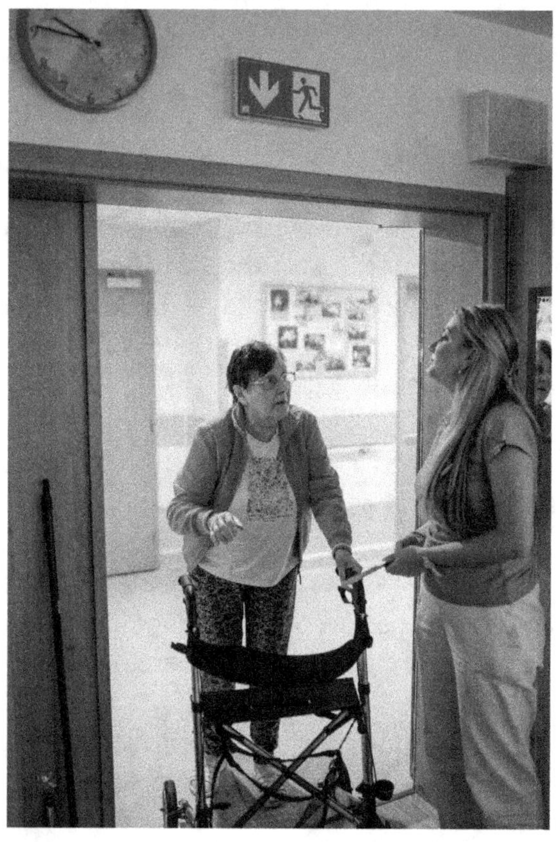

Chapter 1. The Caregiver's Role

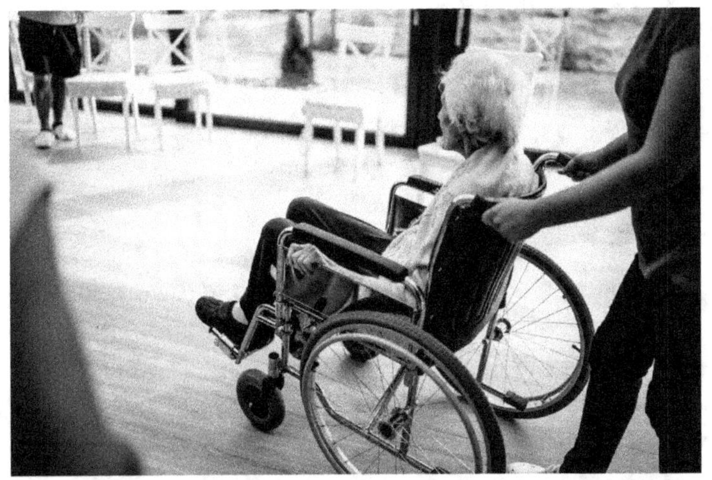

An important factor in a dementia patient's well-being is their caregiver.
Important duties include:

Offering Compassion, Patience, and Understanding: Assisting the person in overcoming their emotional obstacles.

Helping with Daily Activities: As a person's skills deteriorate, assisting with activities like eating, dressing, and taking a shower.

Establishing a Secure Environment: Putting policies in place to guarantee the person's protection and safety, such as house renovations and oversight.

Effective Communication: Creating plans for patient, and clear communication while adjusting to the dementia patient's evolving level of ability.

Monitoring health: This includes scheduling check-ups, taking prescription drugs, and quickly responding to any health issues.

Social life encouraging: As a caregiver you encourage social connections and involvement as a means of preventing isolation and fostering cognitive stimulation.

Acting as an Advocate for the person: Acting as an advocate to make sure that the requirements of the person are satisfied in a variety of contexts, such as legal and medical issues.

Self-care: Realizing the value of one's health and taking pauses to avoid burnout among caregivers.

The caregiver has a dynamic job that calls for flexibility and in-depth knowledge of the particular difficulties that dementia presents. Caretakers make a substantial contribution to improving the quality of life for those suffering from dementia by carrying out these duties.

The Importance of Caregiving

Providing care is an essential and empathetic function, especially for those suffering from dementia.
The main aspects of its significance include:

Enhanced Quality of Life: By providing a comforting atmosphere, caregivers help people with dementia feel more comfortable and well-rounded.

Emotional Support: By offering empathy, compassion, and company, caregivers may lessen the emotional difficulties that dementia patients endure and help them feel connected.

Maintaining Dignity: As people's cognitive capacities deteriorate, caregivers are essential in helping them retain their identity and sense of dignity.

Safety and security: Caregivers take steps to guarantee a secure living environment by lowering dangers and averting mishaps.
Interaction Help: Caregivers may minimize irritation and foster a feeling of inclusion by developing effective communication skills that improve relationships.

Advocacy: In order to guarantee that people with dementia get the proper care and assistance, caregivers fight for the interests and rights of these people in a variety of contexts.

Postponing Institutionalization: Receiving high-quality care may often postpone the need for institutional care, enabling people to live longer in comfortable environments.

Making a contribution to Research and Understanding: Through their active involvement in providing care, caregivers provide insightful information that helps researchers and medical professionals better understand and manage the difficulties associated with dementia.

Emotional and Physical Challenges

Emotional challenges

Providing care for those suffering from dementia presents a variety of emotional difficulties for those providing the care. These might consist of:

Stress and Anxiety: Trying to balance your personal responsibilities and caregiving duties might make you feel more stressed and anxious.

Guilt and Frustration: When dealing with behavioral issues and communication challenges, caregivers may feel frustrated as well as guilty for not doing more.

Pain and Loss: Seeing a loved one's mental capacity deteriorate may cause sadness and a sense of loss.

Isolation: The emotionally taxing aspect of caring may exacerbate social isolation brought on by its demanding nature.

Physical challenges

The physical pressure of providing care may be devastating to the health of the caregiver. Among the difficulties are:

Physical Stress; Helping with everyday tasks, lifting, and assisting with movement may all result in feeling worn out.

Lack of sleep: Chronic sleep deprivation may be caused by irregular sleep patterns and overnight caring obligations.

Health Problems: When caregivers ignore their well-being, it may result in weariness, weakened immune systems, and long-term illnesses.

Financial hardship: Potential job cutbacks and the costs of providing care may also lead to financial hardship.

For the sake of their well-being and to effectively help those with dementia, caregivers must recognize and address the psychological as well as physical issues. Finding help, taking care of oneself, and getting some time off are crucial tactics for overcoming these obstacles.

Self-Care for Caregivers

Providing dementia care may be emotionally and physically draining. By creating a schedule that includes breaks, keeping up a support network, and requesting temporary support when necessary, you may emphasize self-care. Make your health a priority by eating a healthy diet, getting regular exercise, and getting enough sleep. Understand how important it is to ask for assistance, and think about joining support groups for caregivers to get guidance and advice from others. To provide your loved one with dementia with the greatest care possible, you must take care of yourself.

Chapter 2: Creating a Supportive Environment

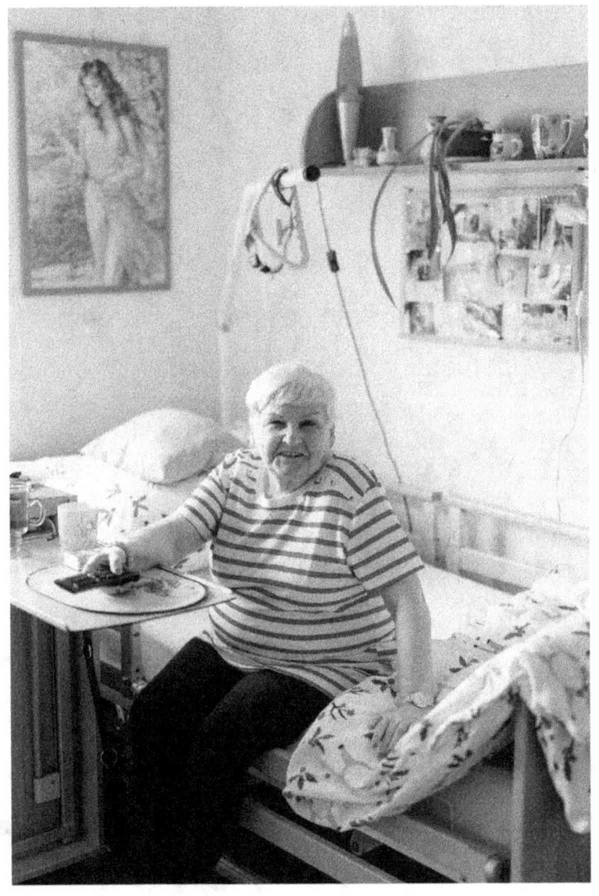

Reducing distractions, keeping the setting familiar, and assuring safety are all important components of creating a supportive environment for those living with dementia.

Establish routines for consistency, promote independence in everyday duties, and communicate in an easy-to-understand manner. Include reassuring elements such as well-known artifacts and calming music.

To help people with dementia feel secure and well-cared-for, cultivate a good environment by being empathetic, patient, and quiet.

Apart from reducing disturbances and preserving comfortable settings, consider adjusting the setting to meet certain requirements. To improve visibility, make sure there is enough lighting, lower noise levels, and use contrasting colors.

Put in place safety precautions including grab bars and the removal of any risks. Add items that are dear to them and beloved pictures to the room to make it seem like home.

Effective communication is essential; use nonverbal clues such as gestures and facial expressions while speaking slowly and clearly. Pay attention to the person's emotions and give them respect. Routines must be flexible to strike a balance between structure and adaptation.

Evaluate the surroundings regularly to adapt to evolving demands and tastes. Work together with medical specialists to include specific equipment or technology that improves the quality of life for the person who is caring for a person who has dementia. A comprehensive approach that takes into account the social, emotional, and physical components of care is necessary to provide a supportive atmosphere.

Adapting the Home for Safety

It's essential to modify the house to ensure the safety of a person suffering from dementia. To avoid falls, remove any potential risks, put in handrails, and fasten carpets. For simple area identification, use color-coded signals and labels.

Make sure there is enough illumination, particularly in the stairwells and halls.

If you're worried about roaming, install locks or alarms on your doors. examine the home environment regularly to meet changing demands and keep dementia patients safe.

To improve safety, think about adopting technologies like motion sensors or smart home appliances. Install grab bars in restrooms to guarantee simple access to necessities.

To reduce confusion, simplify the living area's arrangement and safely fasten large furnishings to avoid accidents. Use familiar furniture and calming colors to create a cozy and peaceful space.

Maintain continuous contact with medical experts to customize home modifications according to the unique needs of the dementia patient.

Family members and caregivers should be encouraged to take emergency response and dementia care-specific safeguarding training.

As the illness worsens, be sure to periodically check and update safety precautions to keep the house a safe and encouraging place. Adapting a house for safety is a continuous process that calls for careful planning, integrating technology, and working with medical professionals.

To improve orientation inside the house, think about adding memory aids like big clocks, calendars, and labeled storage. To make surfaces and items simpler to recognize from one another, use contrasting colors. Install railings along stairwells and hallways if needed to provide extra stability.

When it comes to kitchen safety, make sure everything is taken out of potentially hazardous areas, install automatic burner shut-off systems, and arrange utensils so they are conveniently accessible. Adding text or images to kitchen labels may help with autonomous navigation.

Enhancing Communication with Loved Ones

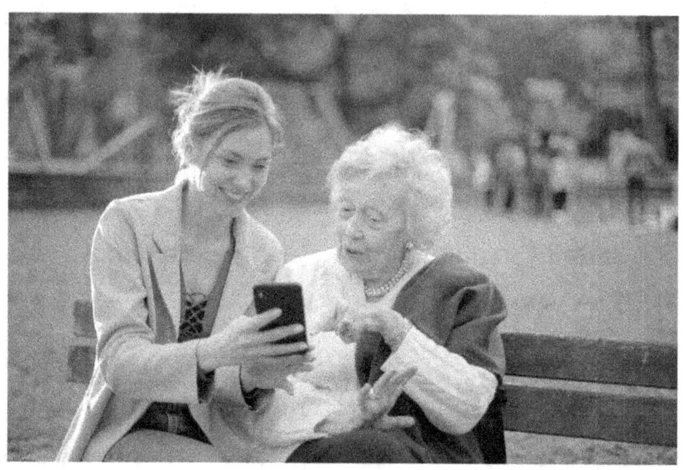

Keep a calm expression, create a routine, and use basic, understandable language to improve communication with loved ones who are suffering from dementia. Use visual tools to help them remember things, such as pictures or memory prompts. Be kind, attentive, and affirming of their emotions. Touch and facial expressions are examples of non-verbal signals that may show warmth and comprehension.

Make adjustments to suit their communication style and provide a distraction-free, encouraging atmosphere. Playing games together strengthens bonds between people and activates brain activity. As their situation changes, evaluate and modify communication tactics regularly.

Include non-verbal clues such as keeping eye contact, giving a soft touch, and speaking in a comforting tone in addition to spoken communication. Make decisions easier and don't give them too many alternatives to choose from.

They feel more safe when you provide a familiar setting with reliable indications. Promote thinking back on the past since long-term memories could be easier to retrieve. It's important to be patient and give them time to assimilate the information and express themselves.

Family members and caregivers should become knowledgeable about dementia to recognize its development and adjust their communication style. Joining support groups may provide both emotional support and insightful information.

Communication techniques should be routinely reevaluated to make sure they continue to work as the person's cognitive skills evolve. In the end, the basis for developing deep relationships with loved ones coping with dementia is keeping a compassionate and understanding attitude.

Promoting Independence and Engagement

Establishing an atmosphere that fosters autonomy is essential to promoting independence and involvement in people, especially those who have cognitive problems. To empower them in day-to-day activities, make jobs simple, and give them clear directions. To improve self-sufficiency, including assistive technology and memory aids.

Adapt activities to their ability and encourage them to participate in things they love. This promotes a feeling of contentment and purpose. Divide up the work into small pieces and acknowledge your progress as you go. Keep up a schedule that provides consistency, since this may help foster a feeling of security.

Respecting their decisions and including them in decision-making whenever feasible are other aspects of promoting independence.

Make the required changes to the surroundings to meet their demands, encouraging independence while ensuring their safety. Assess their talents and preferences regularly so that techniques and activities may be modified appropriately.

In general, encouraging people with different degrees of cognitive ability to become independent and engaged requires carefully balancing assistance and encouragement.

Encourage social connections as well to counteract isolation and improve participation. Make it easier for people to connect with friends, relatives, or local organizations that have similar interests. Engaging in group activities may boost cognitive processes and provide a person with a feeling of belonging.

Provide chances for artistic and musical expression, as well as storytelling, since these pursuits engage both emotional and mental reserves. Exercise that is adapted to their capacities improves cognitive function in addition to general well-being.

A person-centered approach must be put into practice. Recognize their inclinations, passions, and prior encounters and incorporate them into your daily routine. A feeling of identity and self-worth are fostered by this individualized approach.

To provide a dynamic and responsive strategy for promoting independence and involvement, regularly reevaluate and adjust techniques in response to their changing demands. The ultimate objective is to provide a setting that enables people to live happy, fulfilled lives while coping with the difficulties brought on by cognitive disorders.

Chapter 3: Managing Daily Care

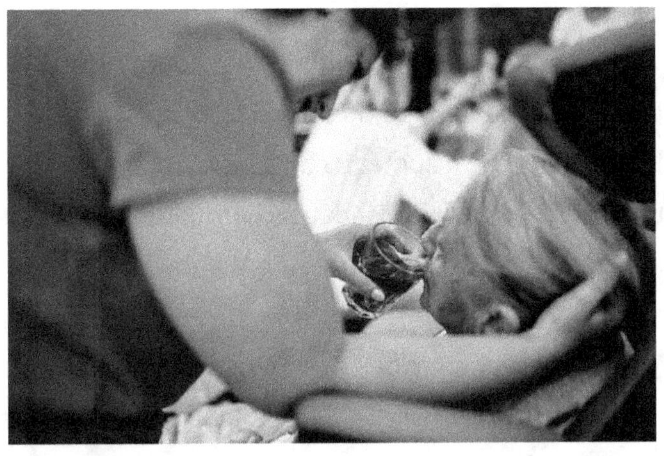

Providing daily care for people with cognitive impairments requires creating a regimented schedule that includes meals, personal hygiene, and medicines. Make things easier, provide polite reminders, and keep the space cozy and secure. It's important to regularly assess your health and communicate with medical specialists.

Participate in activities that enhance your physical and mental health, making adjustments as necessary. Prioritizing self-care will help caregivers be able to provide effective and long-lasting assistance. A routine of daily care that is responsive and compassionate is facilitated by open communication and flexibility in approach.

When it comes to providing day-to-day care for those with cognitive impairments, consistency and patience should come first. To create a feeling of regularity, establish distinct daily routines for things like eating, dressing, and taking a shower.

To improve comprehension, use visual clues and prompts. Continually evaluate their requirements and modify the care plan as necessary. Effective communication is essential; pay close attention, respond to their indications, and provide comfort.

Reduce possible dangers and maintain a safe atmosphere. Work together with medical specialists to address medical requirements and take care of mental health. Providing thorough and compassionate daily care for persons suffering from cognitive problems is based on striking a balance between practical care and emotional support.

Personal Hygiene and Dressing

Self-sufficiency in personal hygiene and independent clothing is essential for those with dementia. Provide gentle reminders, visual aids, and step-by-step directions to simplify the hygiene regimen. Reduce confusion by arranging clothes so that selecting is doable. Wear loose-fitting, comfy clothes with easy-to-fasten fasteners. Foster a feeling of success and encourage self-care by offering assistance only when needed.

Let them feel free to dress as they want, and respect that decision. Evaluate their skills on a regular basis and modify routines as necessary. Furthermore, fostering a relaxed and comfortable atmosphere during these activities enhances the good experience and emphasizes the significance of self-care in day-to-day living.

To improve the experience, use tactile clues such as soft textiles or fragrant soaps. When dressing, provide mild direction, focusing on one step at a time. In order to strengthen their feeling of independence, acknowledge their efforts. Caregivers may handle personal hygiene and clothing routines with sensitivity and understanding if they prioritize comfort and dignity.

Meal Planning and Nutrition

Nutrition and meal planning are crucial to the well-being of people with dementia. Developing a strategic plan entails attending to their requirements while taking into account any obstacles related to meal planning and dietary control.

Create a regular eating schedule first. A feeling of structure is provided by consistency, which makes eating a regular and pleasant aspect of everyday life. Make decisions easier by providing a selection of recognizable, simple-to-eat items. Make sure everything is set up to facilitate meals, including reducing noise and fostering a calm atmosphere.

It is important to take nutrition into account. Choose foods that are high in nutrients and promote general wellness. Speak with medical experts to customize meals for certain ailments and make sure patients get the vitamins and minerals they need.

Encourage people with cognitive problems to stay hydrated by providing water on a regular basis. They could forget to drink.

When preparing meals, put simplicity and safety first. Make use of simple-to-handle cutlery and think about buying premade or readily constructed meals. As far as you can, include them in the process to give them a feeling of ownership and success.

Modify the eating area to increase independence and comfort. Select easily handled plates and utensils. Attend to any sensory issues they may have with temperatures or textures that might affect how they eat. Review food choices and appetite fluctuations often, and modify meal plans as necessary.

Involvement from family and caregivers is essential. Keep up with dietary restrictions by speaking with medical specialists. Work together with those you love to establish a pattern for mealtime assistance. To reduce burden and guarantee consistency in nutritional care, assign roles to others.

Mealtime offers social interaction in addition to nutritional benefits. Promote eating together as a family or group of friends to build relationships. When eating, have a cheerful and patient demeanor and emphasize the pleasure of eating instead of concentrating only on the amount of food consumed.

In conclusion, organizing meals and providing healthy eating for those with cognitive impairments requires establishing a disciplined, encouraging, and pleasurable dining environment. To improve physical and mental well-being, customize the strategy to each person's requirements, place an emphasis on dietary health, and value the social experience of eating together.

Medication Management

Managing medication is a crucial part of providing care for people with cognitive impairments. To guarantee that prescribed prescriptions are administered correctly and on time, a well-organized system must be established. Start by putting together a precise medication plan using resources such as electronic device reminders or pill organizers.

Use visual aids like color-coded labels to make the task easier while identifying various drugs. Together with medical specialists, go over and update the prescription list regularly, making note of any possible interactions or changes. Inform caregivers about the possible effects on general health and the significance of consistent drug administration.

Promote the patient's participation in their drug regimen as much as you can to give them a feeling of control. Explain every step in detail, and if necessary, provide gentle reminders. As soon as possible, address any issues or adverse effects by speaking with medical professionals.

When managing medications, safety comes first. Store prescriptions in a safe place, and discard old or unused medicine regularly. Educate other caregivers on emergency protocols and make sure they understand any unique circumstances about the patient's health problem.

An all-encompassing strategy for drug management is ensured by keeping lines of communication open between medical professionals, caretakers, and the patient. Strive to strike a balance between the therapeutic advantages and possible drawbacks of cognitive problems while evaluating the drug regimen regularly, taking health status changes into consideration.

A complete care plan for individuals with cognitive problems must include successful medication administration, which is made possible by placing a high priority on organization, communication, and safety.

Chapter 4: Dealing with Challenging Behaviors

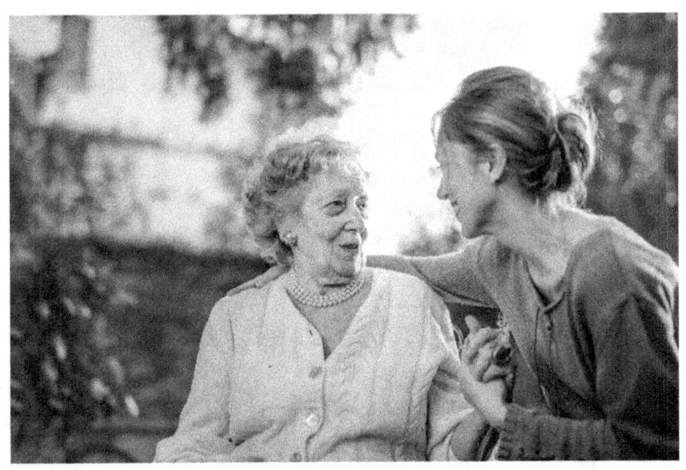

Managing difficult behaviors in those suffering from dementia calls for tolerance, compassion, and a personalized strategy. Recognize that these actions often result from the person's inability to interact with others or manage their environment. Determine triggers using pattern observation and environmental assessment.

Remain composed and avoid conflict when faced with difficult situations. Shift their focus to something better to do or somewhere to be. Nonverbal clues, visual cues, and basic language are all important components of effective communication. Address any unmet needs as soon as possible, whether they are related to bodily comfort, hunger, or a need for social engagement.

Give the individual a feeling of control by including them in decision-making whenever feasible. Establishing a schedule may help to lessen anxiety and problematic behaviors by giving a feeling of predictability. Make sure you have the resources you need as a caregiver to handle challenging circumstances.

It's critical to address difficult habits from a holistic standpoint, taking into account each person's particular experiences and feelings. Reevaluate tactics often and make necessary adjustments, keeping in mind that what works now may not work tomorrow. Caregivers may handle difficult behaviors with compassion by creating a caring and understanding atmosphere, which will eventually improve the general well-being of people with cognitive problems.

To constructively channel energy, and promote meaningful activity and social involvement. The basis for handling difficult behaviors is a compassionate approach that fosters emotional health and reduces stress for both the person being cared for and the caregivers.

Aggression and Agitation

Individuals with cognitive problems may experience unpleasant situations of aggression and agitation, which are often caused by frustration, perplexity, or unfulfilled customer demand. Identifying triggers and modifying the surroundings, emphasized prevention. During episodes, maintain your composure, refrain from conflict, and speak in a non-confrontational manner. Turn focus to relaxing pursuits and make sure you're protected.

Seek advice from medical experts for a comprehensive evaluation and direction on possible solutions, which can include prescription drugs or therapy approaches. Teach caregivers how to spot warning signals and take preventative action.

Managing aggressiveness and agitation requires a comprehensive strategy that incorporates compassion, sensitivity, and expert advice to create a supportive atmosphere for the person receiving care as well as for those around them. Consistent efficacy is ensured by periodic strategy reevaluation.

To reduce agitation, use relaxing methods like soft music or gentle touch. Give them the chance to engage in physical activities to let off steam. Work together with medical specialists to customize interventions to meet the requirements of each patient. Assist in managing and reducing anger and agitation in individuals with cognitive problems by providing caregivers with emotional support and training.

Wandering and Sundowning

People with cognitive disorders often struggle with wandering and nighttime restlessness. Restlessness or confusion-related wandering needs preventative measures like safe spaces and monitoring devices. A regular daily schedule and a peaceful setting are beneficial for sundowning, which is characterized by increasing disorientation and agitation in the evening.

Reduce the amount of stimulants you use at night, provide soothing activities, and make sure the lighting is enough. Take part in mental and physical activities throughout the day to help calm restlessness.

To control and reduce these behaviors, it is helpful to have regular contact with healthcare personnel. This helps create a more supportive and comfortable atmosphere for patients receiving treatment.

Alarms and locks are examples of safety precautions that may be put in place to stop wandering events. To lessen sundowning, create a regimented schedule that includes relaxing activities in the evening. Keep an eye on and make adjustments to the surroundings to reduce triggers, including loud noises or clutter. To control circadian cycles, think about using strategically placed lights and natural light. Work together with medical professionals to investigate drugs or behavioral therapies.

Early indicators must be identified by caretakers, and proper action must be taken. For those dealing with cognitive problems, managing wandering and sundowning may improve their overall quality of life. This can be achieved via a comprehensive strategy that addresses both physical and emotional components.

Hallucinations and Delusions

Delusions and hallucinations, often linked to cognitive disorders, present special difficulties for sufferers and caretakers. Delusions are erroneous beliefs, while hallucinations include seeing things that are not there. It's critical to acknowledge the person's reality and validate their emotions. Reduce any stresses that can cause these sensations by creating a quiet atmosphere.

Avoid arguments and have comforting chats instead. To control symptoms, evaluate drugs on a regular basis and speak with medical specialists. Teach caregivers coping mechanisms, with a focus on empathy and patience. For persons dealing with cognitive problems, a supportive and communicative approach fosters a feeling of comfort while navigating the intricacies of hallucinations and delusions.

Establishing a regular daily schedule might provide stability and lessen the chance of delusions and hallucinations. Take care of sensory issues, including glasses or hearing aids, to improve the accuracy of perception. Create a secure atmosphere by eliminating any potentially confusing stimulations. Work together with medical specialists to determine the root reasons and investigate appropriate pharmaceutical or therapeutic solutions.

Teach caregivers how to communicate with the person by acknowledging their experiences without confirming their own misconceptions. Promote frank communication to learn about their viewpoint, fostering trust and reducing anxiety. Give people coping with hallucinations and delusions thorough, sympathetic treatment by periodically reevaluating symptoms and modifying tactics as necessary.

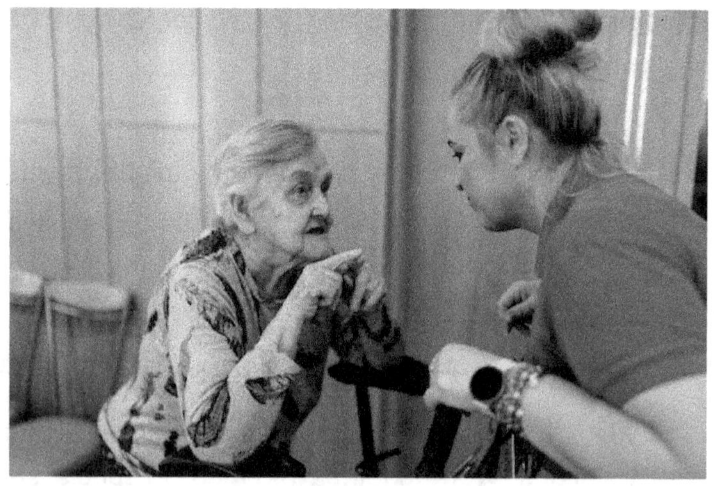

Chapter 5: Enhancing Quality of Life

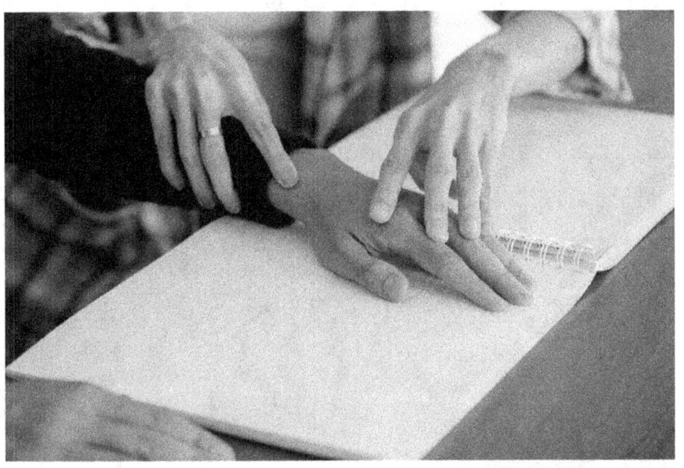

Creating an atmosphere and implementing practices that support satisfaction and well-being are key to improving one's quality of life. It entails creating happy experiences, deep relationships, and a feeling of purpose in a variety of contexts, including caring, personal growth, and community projects. Individuals and carers may strive for a more fulfilling and meaningful existence by emphasizing physical and mental health, social relationships, personal development, and well-being.

Prioritizing emotional support, preserving social ties, and adjusting to changing demands are all important. Completing joyful activities, attending to health issues, and adopting a person-centered approach are all components of a comprehensive quality of life. Developing an atmosphere that supports general well-being requires constant awareness, adaptation, and work.

Meaningful Activities and Hobbies

It is essential to include satisfying hobbies and activities in everyday life to help people feel happy and purposeful, particularly those who are suffering from dementia. Activities that are customized to a person's interests may boost happiness, improve cognitive ability, and provide a sense of purpose. This handbook examines a variety of person-centered strategies for improving life quality via interesting and pleasurable activities.

Engaging in activities that provide emotional and cognitive stimulation includes basic crafts, listening to music, and looking back through old picture albums. Insights on developing customized activity programs, adjusting for changing requirements, and realizing the significant influence of meaningful engagement on the general quality of life for those with dementia will be provided to caregivers.

Socialization and Community Involvement

To provide dementia patients with comprehensive care, socialization, and community participation are essential. Keeping meaningful relationships becomes more important for emotional well-being when cognitive capacities deteriorate.

Recognizing the Significance: Maintaining one's identity and self-worth depends on socialization, which is more than just small talk. Staying socially engaged helps people with dementia fight emotions of melancholy and loneliness. They may maintain a feeling of purpose and belonging by becoming involved in community events.

Adapting Activities to Abilities: As dementia advances, it becomes more important to modify social activities. It is important for caregivers to acknowledge and respect the person's present capacity and preferences. Engaging in basic activities like music therapy, group exercises, or remembering may facilitate social contact without imposing excessive cognitive constraints.

Structured Community Involvement: Promoting attendance at neighborhood activities or dementia-specific support groups helps people feel more connected to one another. These environments foster understanding, lessen stigma, and create a nurturing climate. To find specialized programs, caregivers might look into senior centers, Alzheimer's groups, or local resources.

Overcoming Obstacles: Obstacles could appear, such as discomfort or aversion to unfamiliar surroundings. The trick is to be patient and expose gradually. First, caregivers may start with familiar locations for trips and work their way up to more extensive community participation. Comprehending nonverbal signals and honoring individual boundaries are essential components of effective socialization.

Socialization Has Healing Power:

Socialization is a therapeutic means to some end. Both mental health and cognitive stimulation are facilitated by meaningful interactions, group activities, and emotional bonds. To create an environment where people with dementia can thrive socially, caregivers are essential in promoting these relationships.

Encouraging dementia-friendly behavior:

Fostering a more supportive environment can be achieved through training local businesses, planning awareness campaigns, and creating dementia-friendly locations. Initiations that promote acceptance and understanding can benefit from caregiver support and active participation.

Simply said, community service and interaction are essential components of dementia care that enhance quality of life, not merely optional extras.

Maintaining Cognitive Function

Because maintaining cognitive function directly affects the quality of life for those experiencing cognitive decline, dementia caregivers place a high priority on maintaining cognitive function.

Stimulating Cognitive Activities: Individually designed cognitive activities can increase mental agility and reduce the rate of deterioration. Puzzles, memory games, and storytelling are examples of engaging hobbies that provide mental stimulation and may adjust to changing cognitive capacities.

Including Daily Challenges: Simplified daily chores and challenges can aid in the preservation of cognitive functions. Encouraging people to take part in everyday tasks like organizing, cooking, or making decisions preserves their sense of independence and improves cognitive performance.

adjusting to Changing Needs: Caregivers should modify activities by the recognition that cognitive abilities differ By using a person-centered approach and being flexible with planning, caregivers can provide meaningful engagement that is customized to the individual's present cognitive state.

Promoting Social Interaction: Social interaction improves one's emotional and cognitive health at the same time. Socializing with friends and family, participating in group activities, and having meaningful conversations all support mental health by boosting general well-being, preventing loneliness, and stimulating the brain.

Encouraging a Healthy Lifestyle: Cognitive function is directly impacted by physical health. Promoting a healthy diet, consistent exercise, and enough sleep enhances general well-being. Caregivers are essential in fostering an atmosphere that encourages a healthy way of living and enhances cognitive resilience.

Monitoring Health and Medication: Two crucial aspects of cognitive care are attentive medication management and regular health checks. Caregivers must collaborate closely with healthcare specialists to swiftly address any underlying health conditions that may be compromising cognitive function.

Essentially, preserving cognitive function necessitates various strategy that includes mental exercise, health-promoting activities, social interaction, and attention to general well-being. The purpose of this handbook is to provide caregivers with the information and resources they need to put these tactics into practice and create an atmosphere that supports cognitive well-being for those dealing with dementia.

Chapter 6:Legal and Financial Considerations

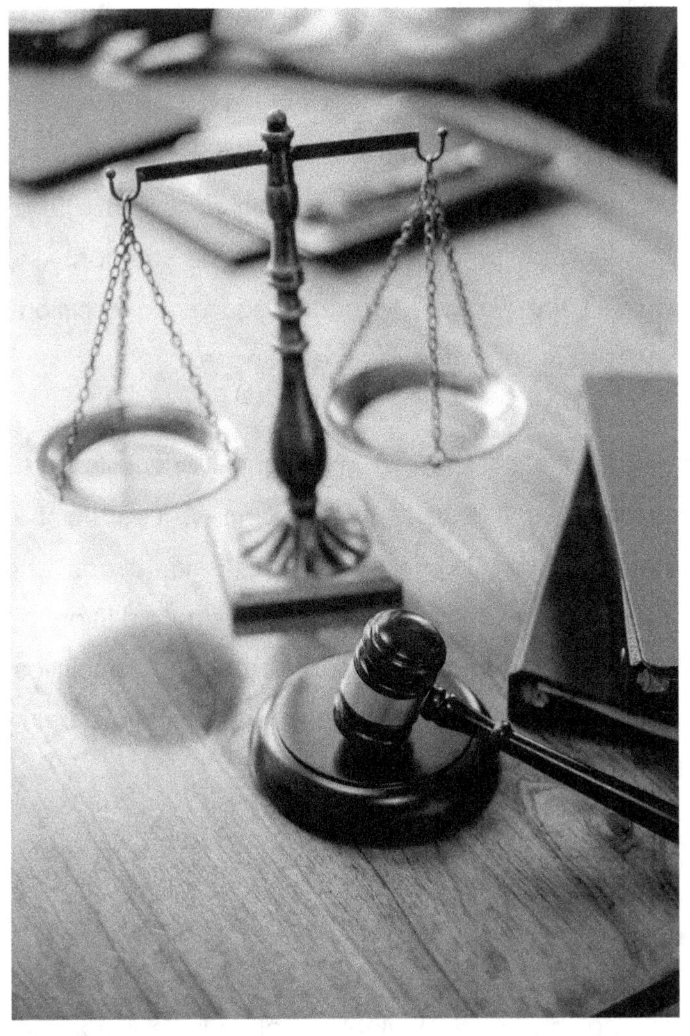

To safeguard the assets of the dementia patient and ensure their well-being, dementia caregivers must navigate the complex legal and financial landscape.

Legal Planning: Creating wills, powers of attorney, and healthcare directives at an early age should be a top priority for caregivers. These legal documents provide caregivers the authority to protect the person's interests and make decisions that are in line with their preferences.

Financial Management: Tight attention to detail is necessary for managing finances. It's crucial to create a budget, look into financial aid options, and keep an eye on transactions. In addition to investigating long-term care funding possibilities, caregivers should exercise caution to avoid being taken advantage of financially.

Healthcare Planning: It's critical to comprehend insurance and other forms of government support as well as healthcare coverage. When it comes to finding the finest available healthcare solutions for a person with dementia, caregivers should take the initiative to do so.

Long-Term Care Considerations: Researching long-term care alternatives and comprehending related expenses are essential. In addition to researching insurance options and weighing the financial effects of various care options, caregivers must prepare for the possibility that they will require residential care.

Caregivers can manage the complexity of dementia care with greater confidence by proactively addressing legal and financial matters. This will ensure the best possible support for the individual's well-being and preserve financial stability.

Power of Attorney and Guardianship

Comprehending the subtleties of guardianship and power of attorney (POA) is essential for dementia caregivers managing legal obligations. A power of attorney gives a designated person the ability to make financial, medical, and legal choices on behalf of a person who has dementia. It's an essential tool for making sure the person's desires are carried out.

When someone is thought to be incapable of making decisions for themselves, guardianship proceedings may be undertaken in court. In this case, a guardian is chosen by the court to act on the person's behalf. Compared to POA, guardianship is a more official, complicated process that requires proof of incapacity. Both procedures come with a lot of responsibility, therefore caretakers should carefully assess the individual's particular requirements and aspirations. They should also get legal counsel to make thoughtful choices that are in the best interests of the dementia patient.

Long-Term Care Planning

One of the most important parts of providing dementia care is long-term care planning, which entails careful consideration of future requirements.

In-home care, assisted living, memory care, and other long-term care choices should all be looked into by caregivers. It is crucial to comprehend the related expenses, insurance coverage, and any government aid. Financial support can be obtained through long-term care insurance, but policy details should be carefully reviewed by caregivers.

It is essential to engage in proactive financial planning, which includes saving money for future medical expenses. Furthermore, keeping up to date on community services and support systems will help caregivers make the best decisions and give dementia patients the best care possible throughout the condition's various stages.

Insurance and Benefits

A vital aspect of providing dementia care is navigating insurance and benefits to ensure complete support for the patient and the caregiver. To ensure that medical costs and future long-term care needs are covered, it is important to fully understand health insurance policies, including

Medicare and supplemental plans. If available, long-term care insurance can play a significant role in reducing the costs associated with specialized care.

When looking into government assistance programs, those with low incomes need to do their research. Along with looking into disability benefits and veterans' programs, caregivers should be aware of the various options available to them for financial assistance. Caregivers must comprehend the intricacies of coverage, eligibility requirements, and application procedures to enable them to obtain the resources they need to improve the standard of care and assistance for dementia patients.

Chapter 7: End-of-Life Care

A delicate yet crucial component of providing dementia care is end-of-life care. Do-not-resuscitate orders and living wills are two examples of advanced care planning documents that should be discussed openly and compassionately.

It is critical to comprehend the person's preferences regarding his or her standard of life and medical procedures. Palliative care can improve a person's comfort level by emphasizing emotional support and pain treatment. Hospice care puts the patient's quality of life above curative measures and is frequently appropriate in the later stages of dementia. Support systems and tools that provide direction on managing the practical and emotional aspects of end-of-life care are essential for caregivers.

Palliative and Hospice Care

Hospice and palliative care are essential in helping dementia caregivers deal with the difficulties of tending to loved ones who are gradually losing their cognitive abilities. Dementia is a multifaceted illness that causes changes in both the body and mind in addition to memory impairment. Palliative care addresses the physical, emotional, and social aspects of sickness to improve the quality of life for patients and their carers.

Palliative care provides relief to the person with dementia and their caregiver by addressing symptoms like pain, agitation, and sleep difficulties. It takes a patient-centered, all-encompassing strategy that takes into account their particular requirements and offers continuous assistance as the illness progresses.

Hospice care, on the other hand, becomes more important as dementia advances and provides dignity and comfort in the last stages of life.

These services, which offer counseling, instructional materials, and respite, are of immeasurable help to caregivers. They guarantee that patients receive compassionate, tailored treatment while enabling carers to negotiate the difficult emotional landscape of seeing a loved one's demise. Palliative and hospice care become pillars of support in the face of the difficult road that dementia provides, enhancing the well-being of both caregivers and their affected family members.

Advance Directives and Decision Making

Advance directives are essential instruments that enable people to express their preferences and decisions regarding their healthcare ahead of time, guaranteeing that their desires are honored if they are unable to make decisions for themselves. A few examples of these legal documents are DNR orders, living wills, and durable powers of attorney for healthcare. They ease the strain of making difficult decisions without clear guidance on the part of family members and healthcare providers by offering a roadmap for medical care and treatment preferences.

When people have a major illness, or cognitive impairment, or are unable to voice their wishes, healthcare decision-making becomes more complicated. This gap can be filled by allowing people to express their preferences for other medical procedures, organ donation, and life-sustaining treatments through advance directives.

This procedure gives people a sense of control over their healthcare future while also respecting their right to autonomy.

In circumstances where people may become incapable of making decisions for themselves, these instructions become extremely important. People can make sure that their values and preferences are taken into consideration while making medical decisions by appointing a healthcare proxy or outlining end-of-life desires. Advance directive discussions facilitate open communication within families and guarantee that medical decisions reflect a person's values, beliefs, and preferences—even in difficult situations.

Grief and Bereavement Support

Compassionate care must include grief and bereavement support, which helps people through the difficult process of coping with a loss. Losing a loved one naturally causes grief, and each person's mourning process is different. Support services seek to provide a secure environment where bereaved individuals can communicate, express their feelings, and find strategies for overcoming the life-altering effects of loss.

There are many different kinds of help available, from community services and support groups to counseling and treatment. Grief-focused mental health providers offer strategies to assist people in dealing with the range of emotions that come with loss, including anger, sadness, and other difficult emotions.

Whether they meet in person or via the Internet, support groups create a helpful environment where people may discuss coping mechanisms and connect with others who have experienced similar difficulties.

Bereavement care goes beyond providing emotional support; it also includes helpful advice on how to handle the practical parts of loss, such as making funeral arrangements and handling legal issues. These programs recognize that grieving is a complex experience, and that comprehensive healing requires attending to both the practical and emotional parts of the loss. Grief and bereavement services offer a lifeline to persons in mourning, helping them through the process of reconstructing their lives in the wake of loss by offering all-encompassing care.

Chapter 8: Resources and Support

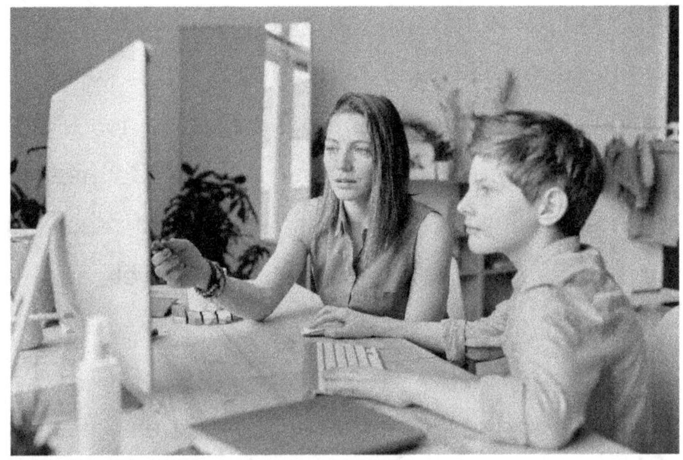

Access to the right services and assistance is essential for the well-being of caregivers for people with dementia, as they face distinct and difficult challenges. Educational resources are essential because they provide knowledge about how dementia progresses, how to care for a loved one, and what support services are accessible. Caretakers can better negotiate the challenges of delivering care by arming themselves with knowledge through online platforms, workshops, and printed resources.

A crucial sense of community is created by dementia caregiver-focused support groups. Through these forums, caregivers can connect with like-minded folks who understand the nuances of caring for people with cognitive decline, share experiences and get helpful advice. Counseling services are also an essential means of resolving stress, sadness, and exhaustion as well as the emotional toll of caregiving.

Helplines and respite care services are examples of practical resources that provide real support. While helplines offer prompt advice and assistance during trying times, respite care gives caregivers brief rest so they can replenish energy.

Initiatives from the government and nonprofit groups frequently work together to offer financial and legal support, relieving caregivers of the load of negotiating intricate administrative environments. When combined, these resources create a thorough support system that recognizes the special challenges associated with caring for a loved one with dementia and seeks to maintain the health of those delivering critical care.

Support Groups and Caregiver Networks

For those providing care for a person with dementia, support groups and caregiver networks are indispensable. These specialized forums give caregivers a much-needed forum for exchanging real-world tips, personal tales, and sympathetic understanding. The difficulties of providing dementia care can be lonely, but caregivers can prevent loneliness by creating a support network through support groups.

These forums help those who are going through similar things by providing a feeling of community and emotional support while also being invaluable resources for navigating the intricacies of dementia care. The combined strength and experience of caregiver networks become invaluable resources for those tasked with providing care for loved ones experiencing cognitive impairment.

Professional Services and Respite Care

The foundations of support for dementia caregivers are professional services and respite care, which provide both necessary relief and useful help. Hiring professionals to help with caring can reduce the strain of providing care, such as in-home healthcare providers or dementia care specialists. These experts provide direction on how to handle difficult behaviors, modify living spaces, and guarantee the security and welfare of dementia patients.

One essential element that gives caregivers brief breaks is respite care. Through in-home respite programs or short-term facility stays, caregivers can tend to personal needs and refuel while their loved ones get high-quality care. This keeps caregivers from burning out and guarantees their physical and mental resilience, which improves the overall quality of care given.

When paired with respite care, professional services provide a supportive framework that acknowledges the particular difficulties associated with providing dementia care and enhances the well-being of both caregivers and the individuals they are caring for.

Online and Offline Resources

There is a wide range of offline and online resources available to caretakers for people with dementia. Online resources include easily available data, online assistance communities, and educational materials to improve caregiving abilities. Websites and forums provide a platform for interaction with a worldwide community dealing with comparable issues. Offline options offer real, in-person support as well as beneficial networking possibilities. Examples include printed materials, workshops, and local support groups.

Online ease and offline community involvement work together to give caregivers a full toolkit at their disposal and create a caring community where they may learn from one another, exchange experiences, and find comfort along the way.

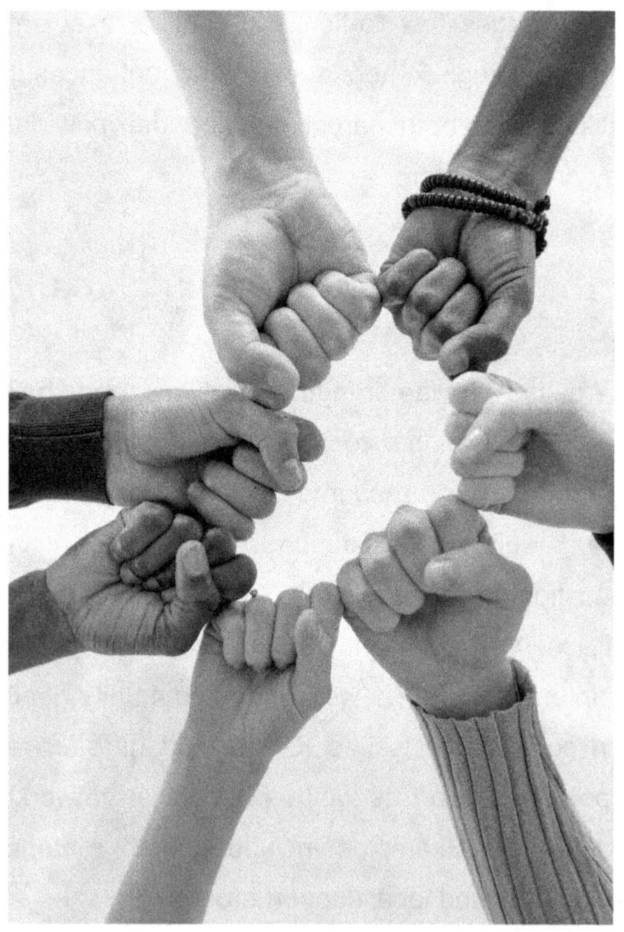

Chapter 9: Conclusion

When it comes to providing care for individuals with dementia or navigating life's challenges, the importance of resources and assistance is immeasurable. These pillars, which range from educational resources to social networks, and mental health services to helpful advice, provide a strong base for people facing difficulties.

The integration of physical and online resources guarantees accessibility and community involvement, promoting adaptability and self-determination. Whether dealing with the difficult task of caring for a loved one with dementia or more general life challenges, there is extensive support that not only offers workable solutions but also fosters mental health. As we acknowledge the significance of these resources, we also underline their vital role in building a society that is flexible, empathetic, and knowledge-based, where people can rely on one another for support and direction when things become tough.

Reflections on the Caregiver's Journey

The path of a caregiver is a fascinating journey characterized by self-discovery, compassion, and tenacity. It's a route that frequently starts off with love and dedication but develops into a maze of difficulties, giving up things and extremely vulnerable times. Caregivers discover strengths they never realized they had when they provided care for others. The trip illustrates the delicate interplay of pain and joy, whether negotiating the difficulties of dementia or overcoming life's unavoidable adversities.

When one considers the caregiver's journey, a variety of emotions come to mind, including the silent triumphs, the unspoken difficulties, the patience lessons discovered, and the poignant beauty found in ordinary, shared moments. It's a path of adjustment, education, and finding comfort in a community that knows the subtleties of caring for others.

When caregivers reflect on the past, they can see not just the difficulties faced but also the opportunities for personal development, perseverance, and deep affection that come with the job. Despite its difficulties, the caregiver's path demonstrates the resilience of the human spirit by creating relationships that endure hardship and the passage of time.

Hope and Inspiration for the Future

The lights that lead us through difficult times are hope and inspiration for the future, serving as a constant reminder that we can overcome adversity and turn it into opportunity. Hope serves as a catalyst in the face of uncertainty, igniting resolve and a belief in better days ahead. It's the belief that difficulties are not insurmountable roadblocks but rather opportunities for development.

Stories of overcoming misfortune and the unbreakable human spirit rising above challenges serve as sources of inspiration. It can be seen in the bravery of those battling sickness, the resiliency of caregivers, and the group's efforts to bring about constructive change. Hope and inspiration drive us to imagine a world where growth, understanding, and compassion are the norm.

Every act of generosity and every demonstration of fortitude serves as a foundation for a future in which people rise to problems together and in which people's capacity for empathy and creativity changes the parameters of what is conceivable. The optimism that we may all work together to create a future where compassion and advancement triumph despite hardship illuminates the path ahead.

CAREGIVERS TRACKER

Weeks	Goals	Remarks
1		
2		
3		
4		
5		

6		
7		
8		
9		
10		
11		

12		
13		
14		
15		
16		
17		

18		
19		
20		
21		
22		
23		

24		
		81
25		
26		

The lights that lead us through difficult times are hope and inspiration for the future

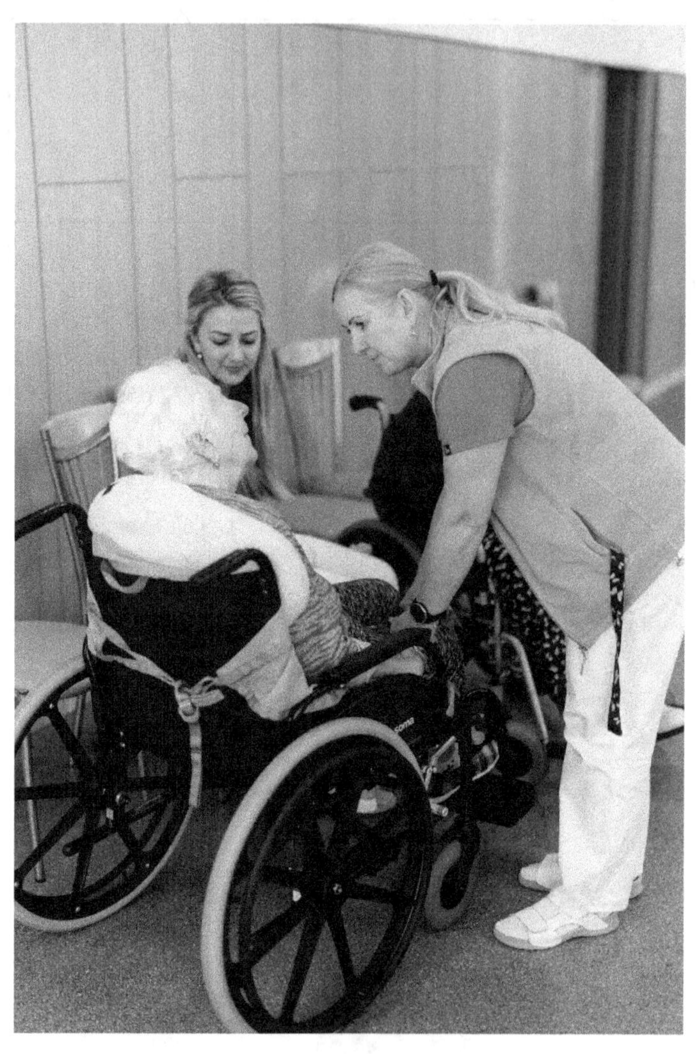